ENDOMORPH DIET FOR BEGINNERS

2024

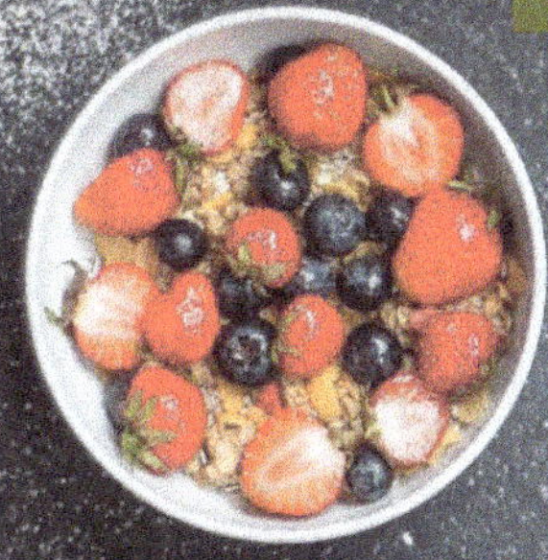

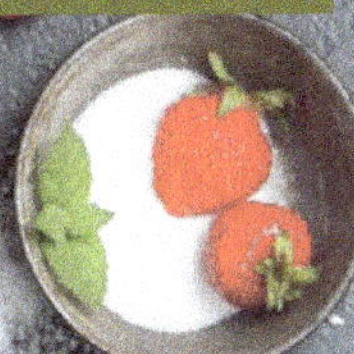

Fuel Your Body, Transform Your Shape with 60 Delicious Recipes and Easy-To-Incorporate Exercises to Activate Your Metabolism

John Milton Doe

Disclaimer:

The information provided in this book is for educational and informational purposes only. It is not intended to replace professional medical advice, diagnosis, or treatment. Always seek the advice of your physician or other qualified healthcare provider with any questions you may have regarding a medical condition.

ABOUT THE BOOK

Dive into "Endomorph Diet for Beginners" and embark on a transformative journey tailored to your unique body type! This essential guide demystifies the science of the endomorph diet, offering practical, straightforward advice to unlock your body's full potential. With 60 delectable recipes designed to fuel your transformation, you'll discover not just how to lose weight effectively, but how to embrace a healthier lifestyle that's sustainable and fulfilling. Expect to learn the secrets of balancing macronutrients, the art of meal planning, and the joy of cooking meals that nourish body and soul. Whether you're new to the concept of body type diets or seeking to refine your approach, this book is your roadmap to a healthier, happier you. Get ready to turn the page on your wellness journey and find inspiration in every bite!

ABOUT THE AUTHOR

John Milton Doe is a seasoned nutritionist and fitness expert with over a decade of experience helping individuals achieve their health and wellness goals. With a Master's degree in Nutrition and Dietetics and a certification in Personal Training, John has dedicated his career to understanding the complexities of the human body and the pivotal role of nutrition in physical health. Specializing in body type-specific diets, he has successfully guided thousands of endomorph individuals through personalized nutrition and exercise plans, leading to transformative health outcomes. An acclaimed speaker and consultant, John's expertise is sought after in wellness circles and professional seminars. His passion for educating others about the endomorph diet is evident in his practical approach to diet and lifestyle changes that promote sustainable health improvements. 'Endomorph Diet for Beginners' distills John's extensive knowledge and experience into an accessible guide that empowers readers to take control of their health journey.

Table of Contents

Dinner Recipes 59

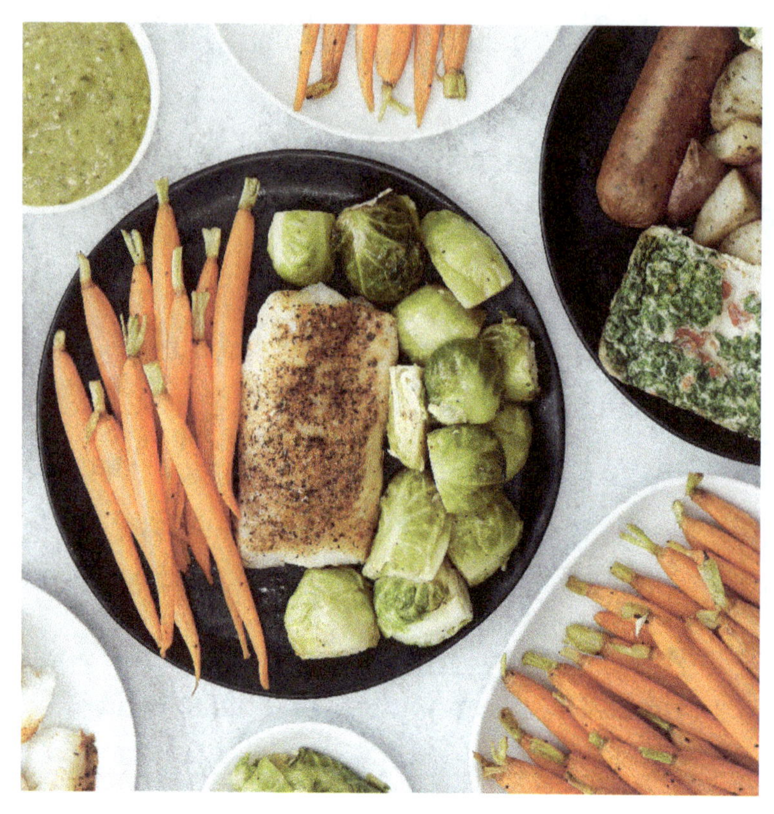

Healthy Meal with Carrots Brussels and Chicken

CHAPTER 1

Introduction

Welcome! Embarking on a journey to better health and fitness can often feel like navigating through a maze of dietary advice and workout trends. For individuals with an endomorph body type, this path can seem even more daunting due to their body's natural propensity to store fat. However, understanding the unique characteristics of the endomorph body type and tailoring your diet and exercise regime accordingly can lead to successful and sustainable results. This introduction to the endomorph diet for beginners aims to demystify the process, providing a solid foundation for those looking to transform their health and body composition.

Endomorph Body Types

The concept of body types, or somatotypes, was introduced in the 1940s by psychologist William Sheldon. He identified three primary body types: ectomorph, mesomorph, and endomorph, each with distinct physical characteristics.

—**Endomorphs:** Endomorphs are characterized by a higher proportion of body fat, a round physique, and a tendency to gain weight easily. They often struggle with losing weight due to a slower metabolism. However, endomorphs also have the advantage of gaining muscle easily, which can be a silver lining when the diet and exercise plan are tailored correctly. Your body type says a lot. Endomorphs, for instance, might find that they cannot eat as much as ectomorphs or mesomorphs without gaining weight and that they need to focus more on certain types of exercise to stimulate their metabolism.

—**Ectomorph:** Ectomorphs are typically characterized by a lean and slender build, with narrow shoulders and hips. They often have a fast metabolism, making it difficult for them to gain weight or muscle mass. Ectomorphs tend to excel in endurance activities and may find it challenging to build muscle despite regular exercise and a high-calorie diet.

—**Mesomorph:** Mesomorphs are often described as having an athletic and muscular physique, with broad shoulders and a narrow waist. They have a naturally higher muscle mass and lower body fat percentage, making it easier for them to gain muscle and lose fat. Mesomorphs typically respond well to both strength training and cardiovascular exercise, allowing them to achieve a well-defined physique.

Endomorph Diet Approach

The endomorph diet is not a one-size-fits-all plan but rather a set of guidelines tailored to the metabolic and physical characteristics of endomorphs. The primary goal is to promote fat loss while preserving muscle mass through a balanced intake of macronutrients (proteins, fats, and carbohydrates), emphasizing whole, nutrient-dense foods, and managing calorie intake. A typical approach includes a moderate reduction in carbohydrates, particularly refined carbs, and sugars, increased protein to support muscle maintenance and growth, and healthy fats to provide satiety and essential nutrients. This diet also emphasizes the importance of meal timing and portion control, critical factors in managing insulin levels and metabolism for endomorphs.

Setting Goals and Expectations

When embarking on the endomorph diet, it's essential to set realistic, achievable goals and maintain healthy expectations. Weight loss and body composition changes take time and consistency. Setting short-term goals, such as improving your dietary habits week by week or increasing your activity level gradually, can lead to long-term success. It's also important to measure progress in ways that extend beyond the scale, including improvements in energy levels, fitness capabilities, and how your clothes fit. Understand that setbacks are a normal part of any journey toward better health and that persistence and adaptability are key to overcoming them.

Nutrition for Endomorphs

The understanding and application of nutritional principles are crucial for the success of the Endomorphs. Here are some foundational concepts:

Caloric Balance: Despite various diet trends, weight management ultimately comes down to calories in versus calories out. Endomorphs need to be particularly mindful of their calorie intake due to their slower metabolism.

Macronutrient Ratio: A balanced intake of carbohydrates, proteins, and fats is crucial. Endomorphs may benefit from a macronutrient distribution that leans more heavily on proteins and fats, with a moderate to low intake of carbohydrates, especially those that are high-glycemic.

While designed with endomorphic body types in mind, this dietary regimen is equally beneficial for individuals pursuing fat loss goals, including mesomorphic athletes seeking to shed excess fat.

To achieve this purpose, utilize these approximation macros.

- o 35% protein
- o 25% carbs and
- o 40% fat

Don't get bogged down by calculations. Simply put, aim for a higher intake of fats and protein while cutting back on carbs. If you find yourself needing sustenance during intense exercise sessions lasting beyond 60 minutes, lean towards protein powder or essential amino acids (EAAs), reserving carbohydrate-rich sports foods like gels and sports drinks for the most demanding activities such as all-day soccer tournaments, marathons, powerlifting competitions, or endurance rides in extreme heat. When consuming carbohydrates in meals, prioritize whole, minimally processed, carbohydrate-rich foods, and moderate your intake of starches and fruits, striving for a 4:1 ratio of vegetables to fruits.

Protein: High-quality protein sources such as lean meats, fish, eggs, and plant-based alternatives are vital for muscle maintenance and growth. Protein has a high thermic effect and can increase satiety, making it an essential component of the endomorph diet.

Fats: Focusing on healthy fats from sources like avocados, nuts, seeds, and olive oil can help maintain energy levels and support cell function without spiking sugar levels.

Carbohydrates: Complex carbohydrates with a low glycemic index, such as whole grains, legumes, and vegetables, should be prioritized over simple sugars and refined carbs. These provide sustained energy and help manage blood sugar levels.

Fiber and Water: A high intake of dietary fiber from vegetables, fruits, whole grains, and legumes can improve digestion and enhance feelings of fullness. Adequate hydration is also essential for overall health and can aid in weight management.

Micronutrients: Micronutrients, including vitamins and minerals, are essential for various physiological functions in the body, such as immune function, metabolism, and bone health. Vitamins are organic compounds that regulate bodily processes and can be found in a wide range of foods, including fruits, vegetables, whole grains, and fortified products. Minerals are inorganic compounds that contribute to structural and regulatory functions in the body and can be obtained from sources such as meat, dairy, fruits, vegetables, and nuts. Ensuring an adequate intake of vitamins and minerals through a balanced diet is vital for maintaining overall health and preventing nutrient deficiencies.

Understanding these nutritional principles and how they apply to the endomorph body type is the first step in creating a diet that supports weight loss and health goals. Tailoring your approach to fit your individual needs, preferences, and lifestyle is essential for long-term success.

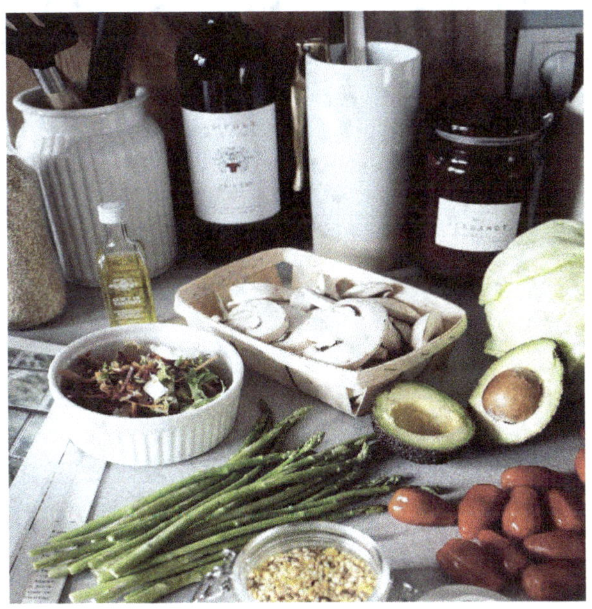

**Healthy Ingredients
Composition of Vegetables**

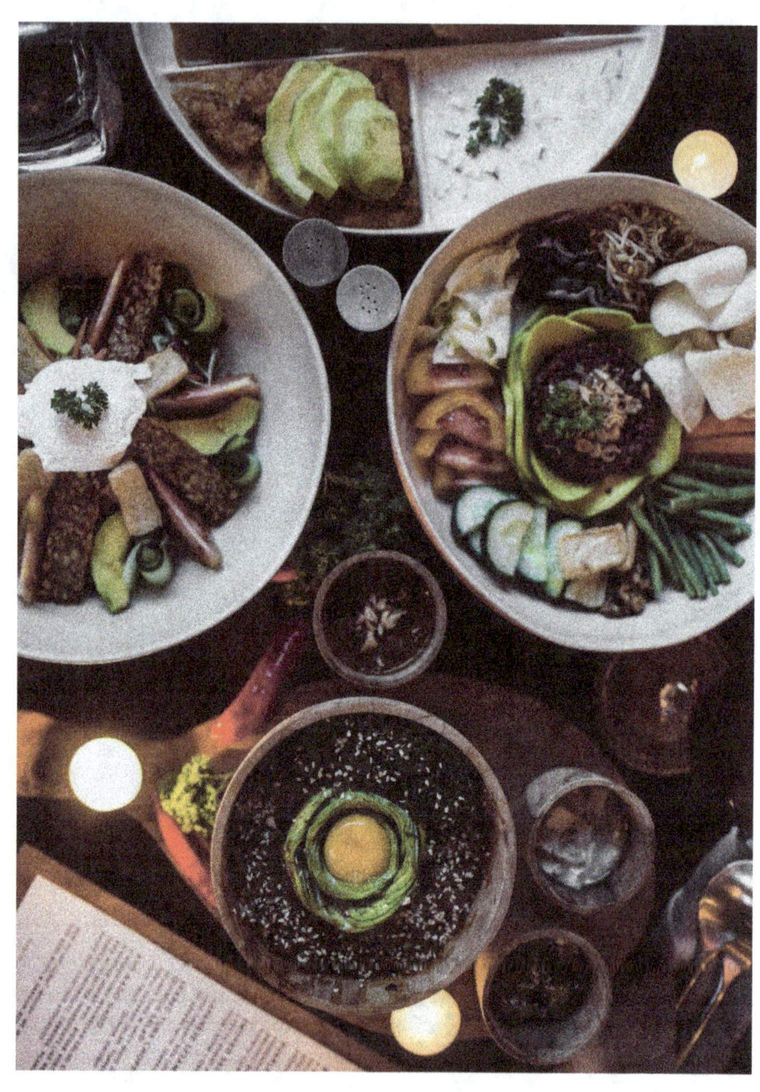

Vegetable Salads

CHAPTER 2

Basics of Calories and Energy Balance

Calories represent the energy content of foods and beverages we consume, and our body uses this energy for various functions such as metabolism, physical activity, and maintaining basic bodily functions. To maintain weight, the calories consumed must equal the calories expended. If you consume more calories than you burn, you'll gain weight, while consuming fewer calories than you expend will result in weight loss. By tracking your calorie intake and expenditure, you can effectively manage your weight and achieve your desired body composition.

Key Principles of the Endomorph Diet

The endomorph diet is tailored to individuals with an endomorphic body type. Key principles of the endomorph diet include balancing macronutrients to support fat loss while preserving muscle mass, focusing on whole, nutrient-dense foods, and managing calorie intake. This diet emphasizes a moderate reduction in carbohydrates, particularly refined carbs, and sugars, increased protein intake to support muscle maintenance and growth, and healthy fats to provide satiety and essential nutrients. Additionally, portion control, meal timing, and hydration are essential components of the endomorph diet to optimize metabolism and achieve sustainable weight loss goals.

Portion Control and Mindful Eating

Portion control and mindful eating are essential components of the endomorph diet, helping individuals manage calorie intake, prevent overeating, and cultivate a healthier relationship with food. Portion control involves being aware of the quantity of food consumed in each meal or snack, while mindful eating focuses on paying attention to the sensory experience of eating and tuning into hunger and fullness cues.

Practicing portion control begins with understanding appropriate serving sizes and learning to measure or estimate portions accurately. This may involve using measuring cups, scales, or visual cues to guide portion sizes. It's important to avoid oversized portions, as they can lead to excess calorie consumption and weight gain over time.

Mindful eating encourages individuals to slow down and savor each bite, paying attention to the taste, texture, and aroma of food. By eating mindfully, individuals can better recognize feelings of hunger and fullness, which helps prevent overeating. Techniques such as chewing food slowly, putting down utensils between bites, and minimizing distractions during meals can promote mindful eating habits.

Developing mindfulness around food also involves being attuned to emotional and environmental triggers that may lead to overeating, such as stress, boredom, or social pressures.

Timing of Meals and Snacks

The timing of meals and snacks can influence energy levels, metabolism, and overall dietary adherence for individuals following the endomorph diet. While there is no one-size-fits-all approach to meal timing, some general guidelines can help optimize nutrient intake and support weight management goals.

One common recommendation is to eat regular meals and snacks throughout the day to maintain steady energy levels and prevent excessive hunger, which can lead to overeating. Aim for balanced meals that include a combination of carbohydrates, proteins, and fats to provide sustained energy and promote satiety.

Many experts recommend spacing meals and snacks evenly throughout the day, typically every 3-4 hours, to maintain stable blood sugar levels and prevent energy crashes. This approach can also help regulate appetite and prevent overeating at later meals.

Some individuals may benefit from experimenting with intermittent fasting or time-restricted eating, which involves limiting the window of time in which food is consumed each day. This approach may help improve insulin sensitivity, promote fat loss, and support metabolic health for some individuals. However, it's essential to find a meal timing schedule that aligns with individual preferences, lifestyle, and hunger cues.

In addition to meal timing, paying attention to nutrient timing around exercise can also be beneficial for endomorphs. Consuming a balanced meal or snack containing carbohydrates and protein before and after workouts can support energy levels, muscle recovery, and overall performance.

Endomorph-Friendly Foods

Endomorph-friendly foods are those that support the goals of the endomorph diet, including promoting fat loss, maintaining muscle mass, and supporting overall health and well-being. These foods are typically nutrient-dense, minimally processed, and provide a balance of macronutrients to support metabolic health.

Some examples of endomorph-friendly foods include:

Lean proteins: Chicken, turkey, fish, lean cuts of beef or pork, tofu, tempeh, eggs, and low-fat dairy products are excellent sources of protein that can support muscle maintenance and growth while promoting satiety.

Non-starchy vegetables: Vegetables such as leafy greens, broccoli, cauliflower, bell peppers, cucumbers, and zucchini are low in calories and carbohydrates but rich in fiber, vitamins, and minerals. They can help bulk up meals without adding excess calories.

Whole grains: Whole grains like quinoa, brown rice, oats, barley, and farro provide complex carbohydrates, fiber, and essential nutrients. They can help provide sustained energy and promote feelings of fullness when included in meals.

Healthy fats: Foods rich in healthy fats, such as avocados, nuts, seeds, olive oil, and fatty fish like salmon and trout, provide essential fatty acids and support heart health. Including these fats in moderation can help promote satiety and flavor in meals.

Fruits: While fruits contain natural sugars, they are also rich in fiber, vitamins, and antioxidants. Choosing whole fruits over fruit juices or sugary snacks can help satisfy sweet cravings while providing essential nutrients.

Legumes: Beans, lentils, chickpeas, and other legumes are excellent sources of plant-based protein, fiber, and complex carbohydrates. They can help promote satiety and support digestive health when included in meals or snacks.

The focus is on basic exercises and endomorph-friendly foods. By incorporating them into a balanced diet, individuals can support their weight loss and health goals while enjoying a variety of nutritious and delicious meals. Experimenting with different recipes and meal combinations can help keep meals exciting and enjoyable while staying on track with dietary goals.

Creating a Calorie Deficit

Creating a calorie deficit is a key strategy for weight loss for anyone, endomorphs inclusive. A calorie deficit is when you consume fewer calories than your body requires to maintain its present weight. This forces your body to use stored fat as fuel, resulting in weight loss over time.

To establish a calorie deficit, first calculate your total daily energy expenditure (TDEE), which is the quantity of calories your body requires to maintain its present weight. This can be calculated using online calculators or formulas that take into account factors such as age, gender, weight, height, and activity level.

Once you have determined your TDEE, aim to consume 500 to 1000 calories fewer per day than your TDEE to create a deficit of 3500 to 7000 calories per week, which translates to approximately 1 to 2 pounds of weight loss per week. This can be accomplished by combining reduced calorie intake with increased physical activity.

Keep in mind that it's essential to create a sustainable calorie deficit that allows you to meet your nutritional needs and maintain muscle mass while promoting fat loss. Avoid overly restrictive diets or drastic calorie cuts, as they can lead to nutrient deficiencies, muscle loss, and metabolic slowdown.

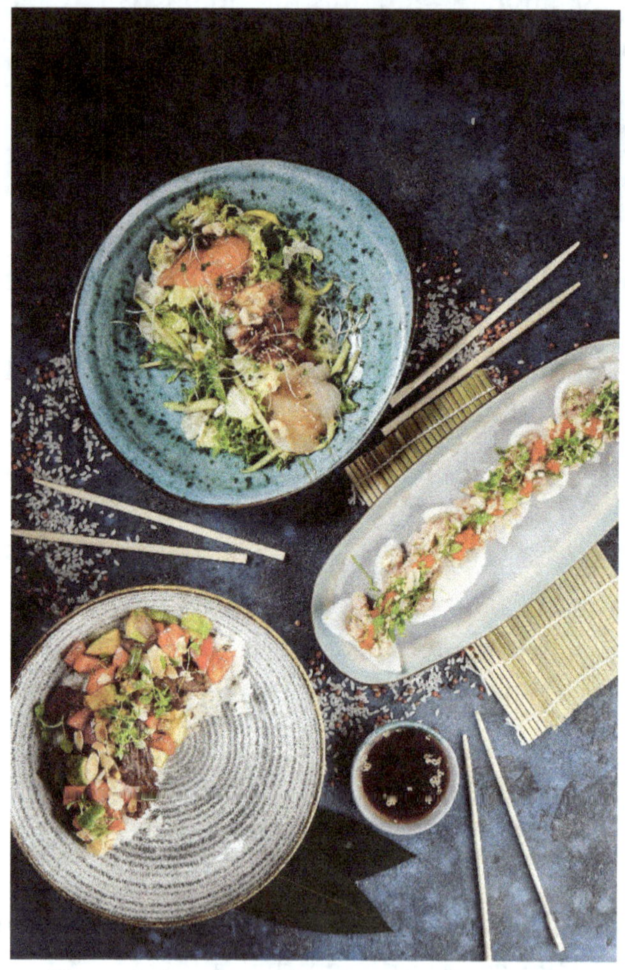

Creating a Caloric Deficit

CHAPTER 3

Effective Exercise for Endomorphs

When it comes to exercise for endomorphs, a combination of cardiovascular exercise, strength training, and flexibility work can be effective for promoting fat loss, building lean muscle mass, and improving overall fitness.

Cardiovascular Exercise

Cardiovascular exercise, such as walking, jogging, cycling, or swimming, can help burn calories and improve cardiovascular health. Target for a minimum of 150 minutes of moderate-intensity aerobic activity or 75 minutes of vigorous-intensity aerobic activity per week, as well as muscle-strengthening activities on two or more days. Cardiovascular exercise includes:

1. Brisk Walking:

- ➢ Find a flat, even surface such as a sidewalk, track, or treadmill.
- ➢ Begin walking at a comfortable pace, swinging your arms naturally.

- ➢ Gradually increase your speed to a brisk pace where you are breathing heavier but can still carry on a conversation.
- ➢ Maintain good posture with your head up, shoulders back, and abdomen engaged.
- ➢ Continue walking for at least 30 minutes to reap cardiovascular benefits.

2. Cycling:

- ➢ Adjust your bicycle seat to the proper height to ensure your legs are almost fully extended at the bottom of each pedal stroke.
- ➢ Start pedaling at a moderate pace to warm up your muscles.
- ➢ Gradually increase your speed and resistance to challenge your cardiovascular system.
- ➢ Keep your upper body relaxed and maintain a steady rhythm with your breathing.
- ➢ Aim for a duration of at least 30 minutes, adjusting intensity as needed.

3. Swimming:

- ➢ Choose a swimming stroke that you are comfortable with, such as freestyle, breaststroke, or backstroke.
- ➢ Enter the water and start swimming at a leisurely pace to warm up your muscles.

- Focus on maintaining proper technique, including rhythmic breathing and efficient arm and leg movements.
- Gradually increase your speed and intensity as you become more comfortable in the water.
- Aim for a swim session lasting 20-30 minutes, or longer if you are able.

4. Jump Rope:

Procedure:

- Grip the handles of the jump rope in each hand with the rope behind you.
- Start swinging the rope overhead and jumping over it as it comes toward your feet.
- Land on the balls of your feet softly, with your knees slightly bent.
- Keep your jumps low and controlled, focusing on maintaining a steady rhythm.
- Continue jumping for 5–10 minutes, gradually increasing the duration as your fitness improves.

5. Stair Climbing:

- Find a set of stairs, either indoors or outdoors, with a sturdy handrail for support if needed.
- Begin climbing the stairs at a moderate pace, taking one step at a time.

➢ Use the handrail for support, if necessary, especially when going up or down steep stairs.
➢ Focus on maintaining good posture and engaging your leg muscles with each step.
➢ Aim for a stair climbing session lasting 10-20 minutes, adjusting intensity as needed.

These cardiovascular exercises provide effective ways for endomorphs to improve their cardiovascular fitness, burn calories, and support overall health. Remember to start gradually and listen to your body, gradually increasing intensity and duration as your fitness improves.

Strengthening Exercises

Strength training is crucial for endomorphs to build lean muscle mass, increase metabolism, and improve body composition. Focus on compound exercises that target multiple muscle groups simultaneously, such as squats, deadlifts, lunges, bench presses, rows, and overhead presses. Aim to strength train at least two to three times per week, gradually increasing the intensity and volume of your workouts over time.

Performing compound exercises that target multiple muscle groups simultaneously is an efficient way to maximize your workout and build strength and muscle mass effectively. Here's a step-by-step guide on how to perform each of the mentioned compound exercises:

1. Squats:

- Begin by standing with your feet shoulder-width apart and toes slightly pointed outwards.
- Engage your core and keep your chest lifted as you lower your body by bending your knees and hips, as if sitting back into an imaginary chair.
- Lower yourself until your thighs are parallel to the ground, ensuring your knees do not extend beyond your toes.
- Push through your heels to return to the starting position, keeping your chest up and maintaining a neutral spine throughout the movement.
- Repeat for the desired number of repetitions.

2. Deadlifts:

- Stand with your feet hip-width apart, toes pointing forward, and a barbell in front of you on the ground.
- Bend at your hips and knees to lower your body, keeping your back straight and chest up, and grip the barbell with an overhand grip slightly wider than shoulder-width apart.

- Lift the barbell with your core engaged, driving through your heels while simultaneously extending your hips and knees.
- Keep the barbell close to your body as you stand up straight, maintaining a neutral spine throughout the movement.
- Lower the barbell back to the ground by reversing the movement pattern, ensuring you keep your back flat and hips hinged until the barbell returns to the starting position.

Repeat for the desired number of repetitions.

3. Lunges:

- Stand with your feet together and take a step forward with your right foot, keeping your torso upright.
- Lower your body until both knees are bent at 90-degree angles, ensuring your front knee does not extend beyond your toes.
- Push through your right heel to return to the starting position, bringing your right foot back to meet your left foot.
- Simply repeat the movement on the opposite side, stepping forward with your left foot.

Continue alternating legs for the desired number of repetitions.

4. Bench Presses:

> ➤ Lie flat on a bench with your feet flat on the floor and your back pressed firmly against the bench.
> ➤ Grip the barbell with an overhand grip slightly wider than shoulder-width apart, arms fully extended, and wrists stacked directly above your elbows.
> ➤ Lower the barbell to your chest by bending your elbows, keeping them close to your body and maintaining a slight arch in your lower back.
> ➤ Press the barbell back up to the starting position by extending your elbows and pushing through your chest and shoulders.

Repeat for the desired number of repetitions.

5. Rows:

> ➤ Stand with your feet hip-width apart, knees slightly bent, and hold a barbell or dumbbells with an overhand grip, palms facing down.
> ➤ Hinge at your hips, keeping your back flat and chest up, and bend your knees slightly.
> ➤ Pull the barbell or dumbbells towards your lower ribcage by bending your elbows and squeezing your shoulder blades together.

> Lower the weight back down to the starting position in a controlled manner, maintaining tension in your back muscles.

Repeat for the desired number of repetitions.

6. Overhead Presses:

> Stand shoulder-width apart and hold a barbell or dumbbell at shoulder height with an overhand grip, palms facing forward.
> Brace your core and press the weight overhead by extending your arms fully, keeping your wrists stacked directly above your elbows.
> Lower the weight back down to shoulder height in a controlled manner, maintaining tension in your shoulders and upper back.

Repeat for the desired number of repetitions.

Tips:

✓ Warm up with dynamic stretches or light cardio before performing compound exercises to prepare your muscles and joints for the workout.
✓ Start with a light weight and gradually increase the load as you become more comfortable with the movements.

- ✓ Focus on proper form and technique to maximize the effectiveness of each exercise and reduce the risk of injury.
- ✓ Incorporate compound exercises into your workout routine 2-3 times per week, allowing for adequate rest and recovery between sessions.
- ✓ Consult with a certified fitness professional if you're new to exercise or have any concerns about performing compound exercises safely and effectively.

In addition to cardiovascular exercise and strength training, incorporating flexibility exercises such as yoga or Pilates can help improve flexibility, mobility, and posture, reducing the risk of injury and enhancing overall well-being.

Building Lean Muscle Mass

Building lean muscle mass is beneficial for endomorphs because muscle tissue burns more calories at rest than fat tissue, helping to increase metabolism and promote fat loss. To build lean muscle mass effectively, focus on the following strategies:

Progressive Overload: Gradually increase the intensity, volume, or resistance of your workouts over time to challenge your muscles and stimulate growth.

Proper Nutrition: Consume adequate protein to support muscle repair and growth, along with a balanced diet that provides essential nutrients and energy for workouts.

Consistency: Stick to a regular exercise routine that includes both strength training and cardiovascular exercise to promote muscle growth and fat loss.

Rest and Recovery: Allow your muscles time to recover between workouts by incorporating rest days into your routine and prioritizing sleep and stress management.

Combating Plateaus and Challenges

Plateaus and challenges are common on any weight loss or fitness journey, but they can be particularly frustrating for endomorphs due to their slower metabolism and tendency to store fat more easily. To combat plateaus and overcome challenges, consider the following strategies:

Adjust Your Caloric Intake: If you've hit a plateau in your weight loss progress, reassess your calorie intake and adjust as needed to create a larger calorie deficit.

Change Up Your Workouts: Incorporate new exercises, increase the intensity or duration of your workouts, or try different types of exercise to challenge your body and break through plateaus.

Focus on Strength Training: Increasing lean muscle mass through strength training can help boost metabolism and break through weight loss plateaus.

Monitor Your Progress: Keep track of your workouts, nutrition, and progress over time to identify patterns and make adjustments as needed.

Stay Consistent: Consistency is key to overcoming plateaus and achieving long-term success. Stay committed to your exercise and nutrition plan, even when progress seems slow.

Lifestyle Factors and Support

In addition to diet and exercise, lifestyle factors play a significant role in achieving and maintaining weight loss and overall health for endomorphs. Consider the following lifestyle factors and support systems:

Stress Management: Chronic stress can contribute to weight gain and hinder weight loss efforts. Practice stress-reduction techniques such as meditation, deep breathing, yoga, or spending time in nature to promote relaxation and well-being.

Sleep Quality: Aim for seven to nine hours of quality sleep per night to support metabolism, hormone regulation, and overall health. Create a sleep-friendly environment by limiting screen time before bed, establishing a regular sleep schedule, and creating a relaxing bedtime routine.

Social Support: Surround yourself with friends, family, or a support group who encourage and support your health and fitness goals. Having a support system can provide motivation, accountability, and encouragement during challenging times.

Self-Care: Prioritize self-care activities that promote physical, mental, and emotional well-being, such as massage, acupuncture, hobbies, or spending time with loved ones.

It is important to address lifestyle factors and seek support when needed. Your weight loss journey is something achievable so do not despair. Remember that consistency, patience, and perseverance are key to overcoming challenges and reaching your goals.

CHAPTER 4

Breakfast Recipes

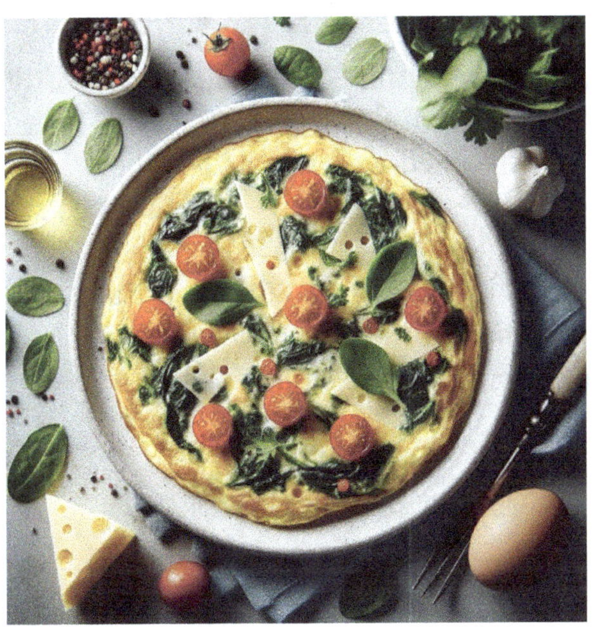

Omelet with spinach and cheese

Ingredients:

- o 2 eggs
- o 1/4 cup of shredded cheese
- o 1 cup of fresh spinach
- o Salt, pepper, and herbs to taste
- o 1 teaspoon of butter or oil

Instructions:

- ✓ In a small bowl, whisk the eggs with a fork and season with salt, pepper, and herbs.
- ✓ Heat a skillet over medium-high heat and add the butter or oil.
- ✓ Pour the egg mixture into the skillet and tilt to spread it evenly.
- ✓ Sprinkle the cheese on one half of the omelet and cook for a few minutes until the eggs are set.
- ✓ Add the spinach on top of the cheese and fold the other half of the omelet over it.
- ✓ Slide the omelet onto a plate and serve hot or cold.

Greek yogurt with berries and nuts

Ingredients:

- o 1 cup of plain Greek yogurt
- o 1/2 cup of mixed berries (fresh or frozen)
- o 1/4 cup of chopped nuts (almonds, walnuts, pistachios, etc.)
- o A drizzle of honey (optional)

Instructions:

- ✓ In a bowl, spoon the yogurt and top with the berries and nuts.

- ✓ If desired, drizzle some honey over the yogurt for extra sweetness.
- ✓ Enjoy this simple and satisfying breakfast.

Quinoa porridge with banana and peanut butter

Ingredients:

- o 1/2 cup of cooked quinoa
- o 1/2 cup of milk of your choice (cow, almond, soy, etc.)
- o 1/2 banana, sliced
- o 1 tablespoon of peanut butter
- o A pinch of cinnamon (optional)

Instructions:

- ✓ In an average-sized saucepan, combine the quinoa and milk and bring to a boil.
- ✓ Reduce the heat and simmer for about 10 minutes, stirring occasionally, until the porridge is thick and creamy.
- ✓ Transfer the porridge to a bowl and top with the banana slices and peanut butter.
- ✓ Sprinkle some cinnamon on top if you like and enjoy this warm and filling breakfast.

Avocado toast with eggs and bacon

Ingredients:

- o 2 slices of whole wheat bread
- o 1/2 avocado, mashed
- o Salt, pepper, and lemon juice to taste
- o 2 eggs, cooked to your preference (scrambled, fried, poached, etc.)
- o 2 slices of bacon, cooked and drained

Instructions:

- ✓ Toast the bread in a toaster or oven until golden and crisp.
- ✓ In a small bowl, mash the avocado with a fork and season with salt, pepper, and lemon juice.
- ✓ Spread the avocado mixture over the toast and top with the eggs and bacon.
- ✓ Enjoy this hearty and savory breakfast.

Smoothie bowl with granola and fruits

Ingredients:

- o 1 cup of frozen mixed berries
- o 1/2 cup of plain Greek yogurt
- o 1/4 cup of milk of your choice
- o 1/4 cup of granola

- o 1/4 cup of fresh fruits of your choice (banana, kiwi, mango, etc.)

Instructions:

- ✓ In a blender, combine the frozen berries, yogurt, and milk and blend until smooth and thick.
- ✓ Pour the smoothie into a bowl and top with the granola and fresh fruits.
- ✓ Enjoy this refreshing and nutritious breakfast.

Cottage cheese pancakes with blueberry sauce

Ingredients:

- o 1 cup of cottage cheese
- o 2 eggs
- o 1/4 cup of whole wheat flour
- o 1 teaspoon of baking powder
- o 1/4 teaspoon of salt
- o 1 teaspoon of vanilla extract
- o 1 tablespoon of butter or oil
- o 1 cup of fresh or frozen blueberries
- o 2 tablespoons of water
- o 2 tablespoons of honey

Instructions:

- ✓ In a blender, combine the cottage cheese, eggs, flour, baking powder, salt, and vanilla and blend until smooth and frothy.
- ✓ Heat a griddle or skillet over medium-high heat and grease with butter or oil.
- ✓ Drop about 1/4 cup of batter onto the griddle and cook for about 3 minutes per side, until golden and fluffy.
- ✓ Repeat with the remaining batter, keeping the pancakes warm in the oven.
- ✓ In a small saucepan, combine the blueberries, water, and honey and bring to a boil.
- ✓ Reduce the heat and simmer for about 10 minutes, stirring occasionally, until the sauce is thick and syrupy.
- ✓ Serve the pancakes with the blueberry sauce and enjoy this sweet and protein-packed breakfast.

Chia pudding with coconut and pineapple

Ingredients:

- o 1/4 cup of chia seeds
- o 1 cup of coconut milk
- o 2 tablespoons of honey

- o 1/4 teaspoon of vanilla extract
- o A pinch of salt
- o 1/4 cup of diced pineapple
- o 2 tablespoons of shredded coconut

Instructions:

- ✓ In an average-sized bowl, whisk together the chia seeds, coconut milk, honey, vanilla, and salt until well combined.
- ✓ Cover the bowl and refrigerate for at least 4 hours or overnight, until the chia seeds have absorbed the liquid and formed a pudding-like texture.
- ✓ In a small skillet, toast the shredded coconut over medium heat, stirring frequently, until golden and crisp.
- ✓ Transfer the chia pudding to a bowl and top with the pineapple and toasted coconut.
- ✓ Enjoy this tropical and fiber-rich breakfast.

Egg muffins with ham and cheese

Ingredients:

- o 6 eggs
- o 1/4 cup of milk of your choice
- o Salt, pepper, and herbs to taste
- o 1/4 cup of diced ham

o   1/4 cup of shredded cheese
o   Cooking spray or oil

Instructions:

✓ Preheat the oven to 180°C (350°F) and grease a 12-cup muffin tin with cooking spray or oil.
✓ In a large bowl, whisk the eggs, milk, salt, pepper, and herbs until well combined.
✓ Equally, divide the ham and cheese among the muffin cups.
✓ Fill each cup approximately 3/4 with egg mixture over the ham and cheese.
✓ Bake for 15 to 20 minutes, until the eggs are set and lightly browned.
✓ Before removing from the tin, allow the muffins to cool first.
✓ Enjoy these portable and protein-rich breakfast muffins.

Salmon and cream cheese bagel

Ingredients:

o   1 whole wheat bagel, sliced and toasted
o   2 tablespoons of cream cheese
o   2 ounces of smoked salmon
o   2 slices of tomato
o   2 leaves of lettuce
o   Salt, pepper, and lemon juice to taste

Instructions:

- ✓ Spread the cream cheese over the bagel halves.
- ✓ Top one half with the smoked salmon and season with salt, pepper, and lemon juice.
- ✓ Add the tomato and lettuce slices and cover with the other bagel half.
- ✓ Cut in half and enjoy this delicious and omega-3-rich breakfast sandwich.

Almond butter and banana waffles

Ingredients:

- o 1 cup of almond flour
- o 2 eggs
- o 1/4 cup of milk of your choice
- o 2 tablespoons of almond butter
- o 1 teaspoon of baking powder
- o 1/4 teaspoon of salt
- o 1/4 teaspoon of cinnamon
- o Cooking spray or oil
- o 1 banana, sliced
- o More almond butter for topping (optional)

Instructions:

- ✓ In a blender, combine the almond flour, eggs, milk, almond butter, baking powder, salt, and cinnamon and blend until smooth and thick.
- ✓ Heat a waffle maker and spray with cooking spray or oil.
- ✓ Pour about 1/4 cup of batter onto the waffle maker and cook for about 4 minutes, until golden and crisp.
- ✓ Repeat with the remaining batter, keeping the waffles warm in the oven.
- ✓ Serve the waffles with the banana slices and more almond butter if desired.
- ✓ Enjoy this gluten-free and nutty breakfast.

CHAPTER 5

Lunch Recipes

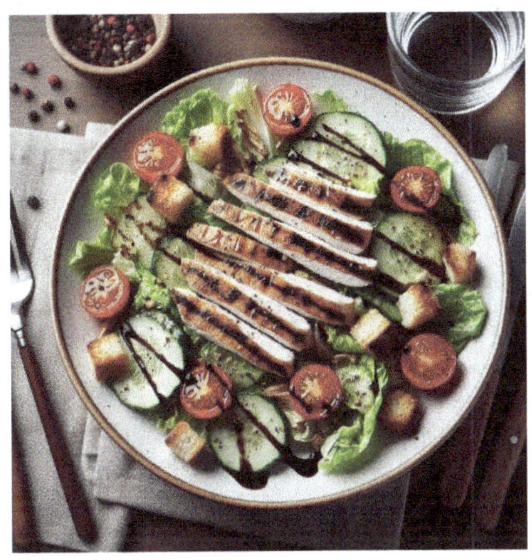

Grilled Chicken Salad:

Ingredients:

- o 2 chicken breasts
- o 4 cups mixed salad greens
- o 1 cup cherry tomatoes, halved
- o 1 cucumber, sliced
- o 1/2 red onion, thinly sliced
- o 1 avocado, sliced
- o 2 tablespoons olive oil
- o 2 tablespoons balsamic vinegar

Instructions:

- ✓ Preheat the grill to medium-high heat.
- ✓ Season chicken breasts with salt and pepper.
- ✓ Grill the chicken for about 8 minutes per side or allow it to cook through.
- ✓ In a large bowl, toss salad greens, cherry tomatoes, cucumber, red onion, and avocado slices.
- ✓ Drizzle with olive oil and balsamic vinegar.
- ✓ Slice grilled chicken and place on top of the salad.
- ✓ Serve immediately.

Black Bean Stuffed Bell Peppers with Quinoa:

Ingredients:

- o 4 bell peppers
- o 1 cup quinoa, cooked
- o 1 cup black beans, cooked
- o 1/2 cup corn kernels
- o 1/2 cup diced tomatoes
- o 1/2 onion, diced
- o 2 cloves garlic, minced
- o 1 teaspoon cumin
- o 1 teaspoon paprika

o   1/2 cup shredded cheese (optional)

Instructions:

- ✓ Preheat the oven to 375°F (190°C).
- ✓ Cut the tops off bell peppers with the seeds removed.
- ✓ In an average-sized skillet, sauté the onion and garlic until softened.
- ✓ Add cooked quinoa, black beans, corn kernels, diced tomatoes, cumin, and paprika to the skillet. Cook until heated through.
- ✓ Stuff bell peppers with a quinoa and black bean mixture.
- ✓ Place stuffed bell peppers in a baking dish.
- ✓ If desired, sprinkle shredded cheese on top.
- ✓ Bake for about 25 minutes, or allow to cook until the peppers are tender.
- ✓ Serve hot.

Salmon and Asparagus Foil Packets:

Ingredients:

- o   2 salmon fillets
- o   1 bunch asparagus spears
- o   1 lemon, sliced
- o   2 tablespoons olive oil
- o   2 cloves garlic, minced

- o 2 teaspoons dill, chopped
- o Salt and pepper to taste

Instructions:

- ✓ Preheat the oven to 400°F (200°C).
- ✓ Gently place and arrange the lemon slices on top of the salmon.
- ✓ Arrange the asparagus spears around the salmon.
- ✓ Drizzle olive oil over salmon and asparagus.
- ✓ Sprinkle minced garlic, chopped dill, salt, and pepper over the salmon and asparagus.
- ✓ Place the lemon slices on top of the salmon again.
- ✓ Fold foil to create a packet, sealing the edges.
- ✓ Place foil packets on a baking sheet.
- ✓ Bake in the preheated oven for about 20 minutes, or allow until the salmon is cooked through and the asparagus is tender.
- ✓ Serve hot.

Turkey and Avocado Wrap:

Ingredients:

- o 2 whole grain wraps or tortillas
- o 8 slices turkey breast
- o 1 avocado, mashed

- o 1 tomato, sliced
- o Lettuce leaves
- o Mustard or hummus (optional)

Instructions:

- ✓ Lay the wraps or tortillas on a flat surface.
- ✓ Spread mashed avocado over each wrap.
- ✓ Layer turkey breast slices, tomato slices, and lettuce leaves on top.
- ✓ Drizzle with mustard or spread with hummus if desired.
- ✓ Roll up tightly.
- ✓ Slice in half diagonally.
- ✓ Serve immediately.

Lentil and Vegetable Soup:

Ingredients:

- o 1 cup lentils
- o 2 carrots, diced
- o 2 stalks celery, diced
- o 1 onion, diced
- o 2 cloves garlic, minced
- o 4 cups vegetable broth
- o 1 can diced tomatoes
- o 2 bay leaves
- o 1 teaspoon dried thyme

    o Salt and pepper to taste

Instructions:

- ✓ In an average-sized pot, sauté the onion and garlic until softened.
- ✓ Add diced carrots and celery to the pot and cook until slightly tender.
- ✓ Rinse lentils and add them to the pot.
- ✓ Pour in vegetable broth and diced tomatoes.
- ✓ Add bay leaves and dried thyme to the pot.
- ✓ Season with salt and pepper.
- ✓ Bring the soup to a boil, then reduce heat and simmer for about 20–25 minutes, or until lentils are tender.
- ✓ Remove bay leaves before serving.
- ✓ Serve hot.

Tuna Salad Lettuce Wraps:

Ingredients:

- o 2 cans tuna, drained
- o 1/4 cup Greek yogurt or mayonnaise
- o 1 tablespoon Dijon mustard
- o 1 stalk celery, diced
- o 1/4 red onion, diced
- o 2 tablespoons pickles, chopped
- o Lettuce leaves

Instructions:

- ✓ In a bowl, mix tuna, Greek yogurt or mayonnaise, and Dijon mustard.
- ✓ Stir in diced celery, red onion, and chopped pickles.
- ✓ Spoon tuna salad onto lettuce leaves.
- ✓ Roll up and serve.

Veggie and Hummus Sandwich:

Ingredients:

- o 4 slices whole-grain bread
- o 1/2 cup hummus
- o 1/2 cucumber, thinly sliced
- o 1 tomato, thinly sliced
- o 1/2 bell pepper, thinly sliced
- o 1/4 red onion, thinly sliced
- o Lettuce leaves

Instructions:

- ✓ Spread hummus on each slice of bread.
- ✓ Layer cucumber, tomato, bell pepper, red onion, and lettuce on top.
- ✓ Top with another slice of bread.
- ✓ Slice in half and serve.

Chicken and Vegetable Stir-Fry:

Ingredients:

- o 2 chicken breasts, sliced
- o 3 cups mixed vegetables
- o 2 cloves garlic, minced
- o 1 teaspoon ginger, grated
- o 2 tablespoons soy sauce
- o 1 tablespoon sesame oil

Instructions:

- ✓ Heat sesame oil in a wok over high heat.
- ✓ Add sliced chicken breast and cook until browned and cooked through.
- ✓ Take the chicken off the wok and set it aside.
- ✓ In the same wok, add mixed vegetables (bell peppers, broccoli, carrots, and snap peas), minced garlic, and grated ginger.
- ✓ Stir-fry until vegetables are tender-crisp.
- ✓ Return the chicken to the wok.
- ✓ Pour in soy sauce and toss to combine.
- ✓ Serve hot over rice or quinoa, if desired.

Shrimp and Avocado Salad:

Ingredients:

- 1 pound shrimp, peeled and deveined
- 4 cups mixed salad greens
- 2 avocados, sliced
- 1 cup grape tomatoes, halved
- 1/2 red onion, thinly sliced
- 1/4 cup cilantro, chopped
- 2 tablespoons lime juice
- 2 tablespoons olive oil
- Salt and pepper to taste

Instructions:

- Season shrimp with salt and pepper.
- Heat olive oil in an average-sized skillet over medium-high heat.
- Add shrimp and cook until pink and cooked through.
- In a large bowl, toss salad greens, avocado slices, grape tomatoes, red onion slices, and chopped cilantro.
- Drizzle with lime juice and olive oil.
- Top the salad with cooked shrimp.
- Serve immediately.

Veggie and Quinoa Stuffed Sweet Potatoes:

Ingredients:

- 4 sweet potatoes
- 1 cup quinoa, cooked
- 1 cup black beans, cooked
- 1/2 cup corn kernels
- 1/2 red bell pepper, diced
- 2 green onions, sliced
- 1/4 cup cilantro, chopped
- 2 tablespoons lime juice
- 1 teaspoon cumin
- 1 teaspoon chili powder

Instructions:

- Preheat oven to 400°F (200°C).
- Pierce sweet potatoes several times with a fork and place on a baking sheet.
- Bake for 45-60 minutes or until tender.
- In a bowl, mix quinoa, black beans, corn kernels, diced red bell pepper, sliced green onions, chopped cilantro, lime juice, cumin, and chili powder.
- Slice open baked sweet potatoes and fluff the flesh with a fork.
- Stuff sweet potatoes with quinoa mixture.
- Serve hot.

CHAPTER 6

Dinner Recipes

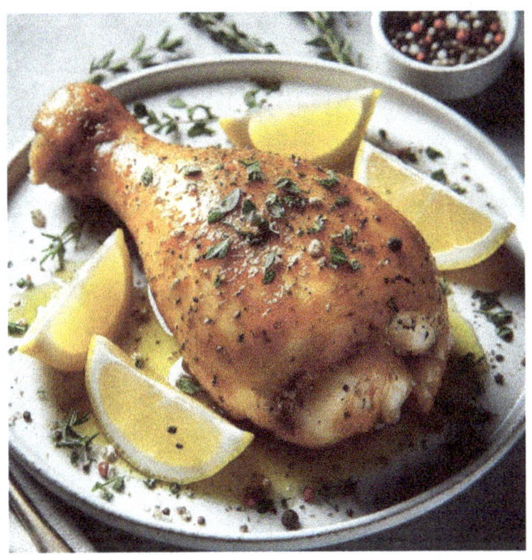

Baked Lemon Herb Chicken

Ingredients:

- o 1 chicken lap
- o 2 lemons, juiced and zested
- o 4 cloves garlic, minced
- o 2 tablespoons olive oil
- o 1 tablespoon fresh thyme, chopped
- o 1 tablespoon fresh rosemary, chopped
- o Salt and pepper to taste

Instructions:

- ✓ Preheat oven to 375°F (190°C).
- ✓ In a small bowl, whisk together lemon juice, lemon zest, minced garlic, olive oil, thyme, rosemary, salt, and pepper.
- ✓ Place chicken lap in a baking dish.
- ✓ Pour the lemon herb mixture over the chicken, coating evenly.
- ✓ Bake for approximately 28 minutes or until the chicken is cooked through.
- ✓ Serve hot.

Garlic Shrimp Pasta:

Ingredients:

- o 8 oz spaghetti or pasta of choice
- o 1 pound shrimp, peeled and deveined
- o 4 cloves garlic, minced
- o 2 tablespoons olive oil
- o 1/4 cup fresh parsley, chopped
- o Salt and pepper to taste

Instructions:

- ✓ Cook pasta according to package instructions. Drain and set aside.

- ✓ In an average-sized skillet, heat olive oil over medium heat.
- ✓ Add minced garlic and cook until fragrant.
- ✓ To the skillet, add the shrimp and cook until pink and cooked through.
- ✓ Toss cooked pasta with shrimp and garlic.
- ✓ Season with salt and pepper.
- ✓ Sprinkle chopped parsley over the pasta.
- ✓ Serve hot.

Vegetable and Chickpea Curry:

Ingredients:

- o 1 tablespoon olive oil
- o 1 onion, diced
- o 2 cloves garlic, minced
- o 2 teaspoons curry powder
- o 1 teaspoon ground cumin
- o 1 teaspoon ground coriander
- o 1/2 teaspoon turmeric
- o 1 can (approximately 15 oz) chickpeas, drained and rinsed
- o 1 can (14 oz) diced tomatoes
- o 1 cup vegetable broth
- o 2 cups mixed vegetables (such as cauliflower, bell peppers, carrots)
- o Salt and pepper to taste

Instructions:

- ✓ Heat olive oil in an average-sized pot over medium heat.
- ✓ Add diced onion and minced garlic. Cook until softened.
- ✓ Stir in curry powder, cumin, coriander, and turmeric. Cook for 1-2 minutes until fragrant.
- ✓ Add chickpeas, diced tomatoes, vegetable broth, and mixed vegetables to the pot. Season with salt and pepper.
- ✓ Gently bring to a simmer and cook for about 18 minutes until vegetables are tender.
- ✓ Serve hot with rice or naan bread.

Eggplant Parmesan:

Ingredients:

- o 1 large eggplant, sliced into rounds
- o 2 eggs, beaten
- o 1 cup breadcrumbs
- o 1 cup marinara sauce
- o 1 cup shredded mozzarella cheese
- o 1/4 cup grated Parmesan cheese
- o Fresh basil leaves for garnish

Instructions:

- ✓ Preheat oven to 375°F (190°C).
- ✓ Dip the eggplant slices into the beaten eggs, ensuring they are fully coated. Then, coat the eggplant slices with breadcrumbs, covering them evenly.
- ✓ Place coated eggplant slices on a baking sheet lined with parchment paper.
- ✓ Bake for approximately 22 minutes or until golden brown and crispy.
- ✓ In a baking dish, gently spread a layer of marinara sauce.
- ✓ Arrange baked eggplant slices on top of the sauce.
- ✓ Sprinkle shredded mozzarella and grated Parmesan cheese over the eggplant.
- ✓ Bake for an additional 15-20 minutes or until cheese is melted and bubbly.
- ✓ Garnish with fresh basil leaves before serving.

Turkey Meatballs with Zucchini Noodles:

Ingredients:

- o 1 pound ground turkey
- o 1/4 cup breadcrumbs

- 1 egg
- 2 cloves garlic, minced
- 1 teaspoon Italian seasoning
- Salt and pepper to taste
- 4 zucchinis, spiralized into noodles
- 1 cup marinara sauce
- Fresh basil leaves for garnish

Instructions:

- Preheat the oven to 375°F (190°C).
- In a bowl, mix ground turkey, breadcrumbs, eggs, minced garlic, Italian seasoning, salt, and pepper.
- Gently shape the mixture into meatballs and place them on a baking sheet lined with parchment paper.
- Bake meatballs for 20–25 minutes or until cooked through.
- In a skillet, heat the marinara sauce over medium heat.
- Add the zucchini noodles to the skillet and cook until tender.
- Serve turkey meatballs over zucchini noodles.
- Garnish with fresh basil leaves before serving.

Stuffed Portobello Mushrooms:

Ingredients:

- o   4 large portobello mushrooms
- o   1 cup quinoa, cooked
- o   1 cup spinach, chopped
- o   1/2 cup sun-dried tomatoes, chopped
- o   1/4 cup pine nuts
- o   2 cloves garlic, minced
- o   1/4 cup grated Parmesan cheese
- o   Salt and pepper to taste

Instructions:

- ✓ Preheat oven to 375°F (190°C).
- ✓ Remove stems from portobello mushrooms and scoop out the gills.
- ✓ In a bowl, mix together cooked quinoa, chopped spinach, sun-dried tomatoes, pine nuts, minced garlic, grated Parmesan cheese, salt, and pepper.
- ✓ Stuff each portobello mushroom with the quinoa mixture.
- ✓ Place stuffed mushrooms on a baking sheet lined with parchment paper.
- ✓ Bake for an approximate time of 25 minutes or until mushrooms are tender.
- ✓ Serve hot.

Baked Teriyaki Chicken:

Ingredients:

- o 4 chicken breasts
- o 1/2 cup soy sauce
- o 1/4 cup honey
- o 2 cloves garlic, minced
- o 1 teaspoon ginger, grated
- o 1 tablespoon sesame seeds
- o Sliced green onions for garnish

Instructions:

- ✓ Preheat the oven to 375°F (190°C).
- ✓ In a bowl, whisk together soy sauce, honey, minced garlic, and grated ginger to make the teriyaki sauce.
- ✓ Place chicken breasts in a baking dish.
- ✓ Pour teriyaki sauce over the chicken, coating it evenly.
- ✓ Sprinkle sesame seeds over the chicken.
- ✓ Bake for half an hour or until the chicken is cooked through.
- ✓ Garnish with sliced green onions before serving.

Moroccan Chickpea Tagine:

Ingredients:

- 2 tablespoons olive oil
- 1 onion, diced
- 2 cloves garlic, minced
- 1 teaspoon ground cumin
- 1 teaspoon ground coriander
- 1/2 teaspoon ground cinnamon
- 1/4 teaspoon ground turmeric
- 1 can (approximately 15 oz) chickpeas, drained and rinsed
- 1 can (14 oz) diced tomatoes
- 1 cup vegetable broth
- 1/4 cup dried apricots, chopped
- 1/4 cup chopped fresh cilantro

Instructions:

- Heat the olive oil in a tagine or large pot over medium heat.
- Add diced onion and minced garlic. Cook until softened.
- Stir in ground cumin, ground coriander, ground cinnamon, and ground turmeric. Cook for 1-2 minutes until fragrant.
- Add chickpeas, diced tomatoes, vegetable broth, and chopped dried apricots to the pot.

- ✓ Bring to a simmer and cook for 20-25 minutes.
- ✓ Garnish with chopped fresh cilantro before serving.

Thai Peanut Chicken Lettuce Wraps:

Ingredients:

- o 1 pound chicken breast, cooked and shredded
- o 1/4 cup peanut butter
- o 2 tablespoons soy sauce
- o 1 tablespoon honey
- o 1 tablespoon lime juice
- o 1 teaspoon Sriracha sauce (optional)
- o 1/4 cup chopped peanuts
- o Lettuce leaves for wrapping
- o Shredded carrots and sliced cucumbers for garnish

Instructions:

- ✓ In a small saucepan, heat peanut butter, soy sauce, honey, lime juice, and Sriracha sauce over low heat until smooth and well combined.
- ✓ Add cooked and shredded chicken to the saucepan. Stir to coat the chicken with the peanut sauce.

- ✓ Spoon chicken mixture onto lettuce leaves.
- ✓ Garnish with shredded carrots, sliced cucumbers, and chopped peanuts.
- ✓ Roll up and serve.

Salmon and Asparagus Foil Packs:

Ingredients:

- o 2 salmon fillets
- o some pound asparagus spears, trimmed
- o 2-4 lemons, sliced
- o 4 cloves garlic, minced
- o 2 tablespoons olive oil
- o Salt and pepper to taste

Instructions:

- ✓ Preheat the oven to 400°F (200°C).
- ✓ Place every salmon fillet on a piece of aluminum foil.
- ✓ Divide asparagus spears equally among the foil packs, arranging them next to the salmon.
- ✓ Place lemon slices on top of the salmon and asparagus.
- ✓ In a small bowl, whisk together minced garlic, olive oil, salt, and pepper.
- ✓ Drizzle the garlic oil mixture over the salmon and asparagus.

- ✓ Fold the edges of the foil to create packets, sealing tightly.
- ✓ Place foil packs on a baking sheet and bake for 15-20 minutes or until salmon is cooked through.
- ✓ Serve hot.

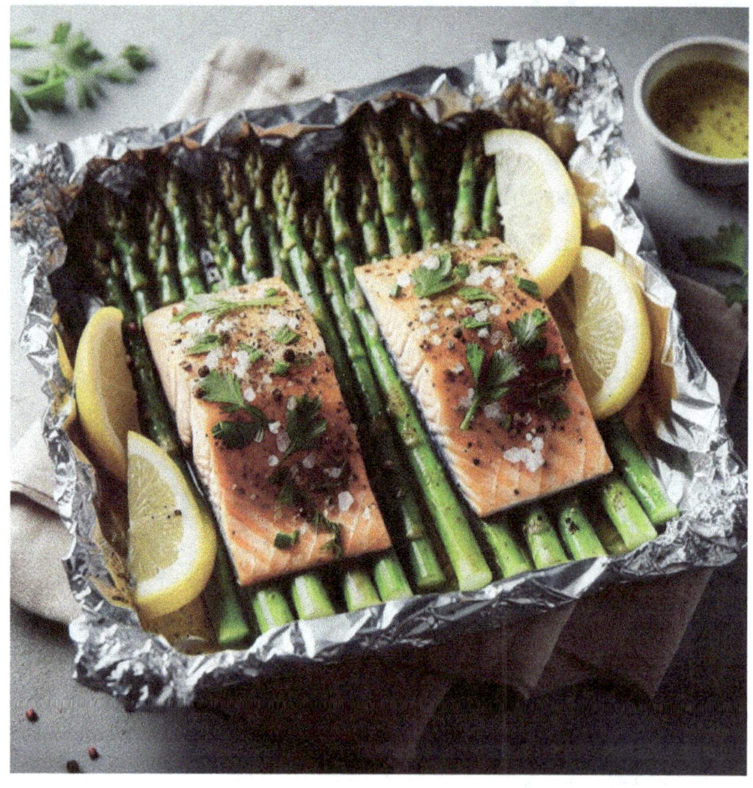

Salmon and Asparagus Foil Packs:

<h1 style="text-align:center">CHAPTER 7</h1>

Desert Recipes

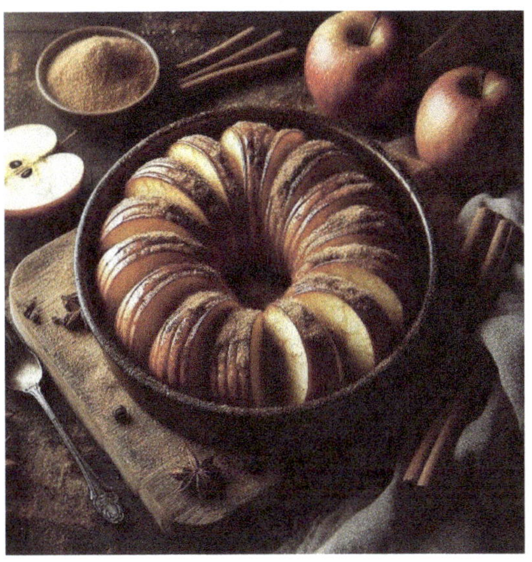

Baked Apples with Cinnamon:

Ingredients:

- o 4 apples
- o 2 tablespoons butter or coconut oil
- o 2 tablespoons honey or maple syrup
- o 1 teaspoon ground cinnamon
- o 1/4 cup chopped nuts (such as walnuts or pecans)

Instructions:

- ✓ Preheat the oven to 375°F (190°C).
- ✓ Core the apples and place them in a baking dish.
- ✓ In a small bowl, mix butter or coconut oil, honey or maple syrup, and ground cinnamon.
- ✓ Carefully spoon the mixture into the center of each apple.
- ✓ Bake for an average of 25–30 minutes or until apples are tender.
- ✓ Sprinkle chopped nuts over baked apples before serving.
- ✓ Serve warm.

Banana Oatmeal Cookies:

Ingredients:

- o 2 ripe bananas, mashed
- o 1 cup rolled oats
- o 1/4 cup chopped nuts (such as almonds or walnuts)
- o 1/4 cup raisins or dried cranberries
- o 1 teaspoon ground cinnamon

Instructions:

- ✓ Preheat the oven to 350°F (175°C).

- ✓ In a bowl, combine mashed bananas, rolled oats, chopped nuts, raisins or dried cranberries, and ground cinnamon.
- ✓ Mix until well combined.
- ✓ Gently drop spoonful of the mixture onto a baking sheet lined with parchment paper.
- ✓ Using the back of a spoon, flatten each cookie.
- ✓ Bake for an average of 12 minutes or until the cookies are golden brown.
- ✓ Allow the cookies to cool before serving.
- ✓ Serve at room temperature.

Dark Chocolate Avocado Mousse:

Ingredients:

- o 2 ripe avocados
- o 1/4 cup cocoa powder
- o 1/4 cup honey or maple syrup
- o 1 teaspoon vanilla extract

Instructions:

- ✓ Carefully scoop the flesh of the avocados into a food processor or blender.
- ✓ Add cocoa powder, honey or maple syrup, and vanilla extract.
- ✓ Blend until smooth and creamy.
- ✓ Taste and adjust sweetness.

- ✓ Transfer the mousse into serving bowls.
- ✓ Refrigerate for an average of half an hour before serving.
- ✓ Serve chilled, optionally topped with fresh berries or shredded coconut.

Coconut Mango Sorbet:

Ingredients:

- o 2 cups frozen mango chunks
- o 1/2 cup coconut milk
- o 2 tablespoons honey or maple syrup
- o 1 tablespoon lime juice

Instructions:

- ✓ In a blender, combine frozen mango chunks, coconut milk, honey or maple syrup, and lime juice.
- ✓ Blend until smooth and creamy.
- ✓ Taste and adjust sweetness.
- ✓ Transfer the sorbet mixture to a shallow dish.
- ✓ Freeze for not less than 2 hours or until firm.
- ✓ Give some time for the sorbet to soften slightly at room temperature before serving.
- ✓ Serve chilled, optionally garnished with fresh mint leaves.

Almond Flour Banana Bread:

Ingredients:

- 2 ripe bananas, mashed
- 2 eggs
- 1/4 cup coconut oil, melted
- 1/4 cup honey or maple syrup
- 1 teaspoon vanilla extract
- 2 cups almond flour
- 1 teaspoon baking powder
- 1/2 teaspoon ground cinnamon

Instructions:

- Preheat the oven to 350°F (175°C). Grease a loaf pan with coconut oil.
- In a large bowl, whisk together mashed bananas, eggs, melted coconut oil, honey or maple syrup, and vanilla extract.
- In a separate bowl, combine the almond flour, baking powder, and ground cinnamon.
- Carefully and slowly add the dry ingredients to the wet ingredients, stirring until well combined.
- Gently pour the batter into the prepared loaf pan.

- ✓ Bake for an average of 45 minutes or until a toothpick inserted into the center comes out clean.
- ✓ Allow banana bread to cool in the pan for 10 minutes before transferring it to a wire rack to cool completely.
- ✓ Slice and serve.

Protein-Packed Chocolate Peanut Butter Balls:

Ingredients:

- o 1 cup rolled oats
- o 1/2 cup natural peanut butter
- o 1/4 cup honey or maple syrup
- o 1/4 cup chocolate protein powder
- o 1/4 cup mini chocolate chips

Instructions:

- ✓ In a large bowl, mix rolled oats, peanut butter, honey or maple syrup, chocolate protein powder, and mini chocolate chips until well combined.
- ✓ Carefully roll the mixture into balls using your hands.
- ✓ Gently place the balls on a baking sheet lined with parchment paper.

✓ Refrigerate for 30 minutes to set.
✓ Serve chilled.

Baked Pears with Cinnamon and Walnuts:

Ingredients:

o 4 ripe pears, halved and cored
o 1 tablespoon coconut oil, melted
o 2 tablespoons honey or maple syrup
o 1 teaspoon ground cinnamon
o 1/4 cup chopped walnuts

Instructions:

✓ Preheat the oven to 375°F (190°C).
✓ Carefully place pear halves, cut side up, in a baking dish.
✓ In a small bowl, mix together melted coconut oil, honey or maple syrup, and ground cinnamon.
✓ Drizzle the mixture over the pear halves.
✓ Sprinkle chopped walnuts on top.
✓ Bake for 25-30 minutes or until pears are tender.
✓ Serve warm.

Raspberry Chia Jam:

Ingredients:

- o   2 cups fresh raspberries
- o   2 tablespoons honey or maple syrup
- o   2 tablespoons chia seeds

Instructions:

- ✓ In a saucepan, heat raspberries and honey or maple syrup over medium heat.
- ✓ Cook until raspberries break down and release their juices, stirring occasionally.
- ✓ Mash the raspberries with a fork or potato masher.
- ✓ Stir in the chia seeds and continue to cook for another 5 minutes, stirring constantly.
- ✓ Take it away from the heat and let the jam cool.
- ✓ Transfer the jam to a jar and refrigerate until ready to use.
- ✓ Serve chilled.

Cinnamon Baked Pear Chips:

Ingredients:

- o   2 ripe pears
- o   1 teaspoon ground cinnamon

Instructions:

- ✓ Preheat oven to 225°F (110°C). Line a baking sheet with parchment paper.
- ✓ Thinly slice the pears crosswise, discarding the seeds.
- ✓ Place the pear slices in a single layer on the prepared baking sheet.
- ✓ Sprinkle ground cinnamon over the pear slices.
- ✓ Bake for 1.5-2 hours or until the pear chips are dried and slightly crispy.
- ✓ Let the pear chips cool completely before serving.
- ✓ Serve at room temperature.

Lemon Poppy Seed Muffins:

Ingredients:

- o 2 cups almond flour
- o 1/4 cup coconut flour
- o 1/4 cup coconut sugar
- o 1 tablespoon poppy seeds
- o 1 teaspoon baking powder
- o 1/2 teaspoon baking soda
- o Pinch of salt
- o 1/2 cup unsweetened almond milk

- o 1/4 cup coconut oil, melted
- o 2 eggs
- o Zest and juice of 1 lemon
- o 1 teaspoon vanilla extract

Instructions:

- ✓ Preheat the oven to 350°F (175°C). Line a muffin tin with paper liners.
- ✓ In a large bowl, whisk together almond flour, coconut flour, coconut sugar, poppy seeds, baking powder, baking soda, and salt.
- ✓ In another bowl, whisk together almond milk, melted coconut oil, eggs, lemon zest, lemon juice, and vanilla extract.
- ✓ Add the wet ingredients to the dry ingredients and mix just until combined.
- ✓ Split the batter evenly into the muffin cups.
- ✓ Bake for an average of 20 minutes or until a toothpick inserted into the center comes out clean.
- ✓ Let the muffins cool before serving.

CHAPTER 8

Snacks and Side Dishes

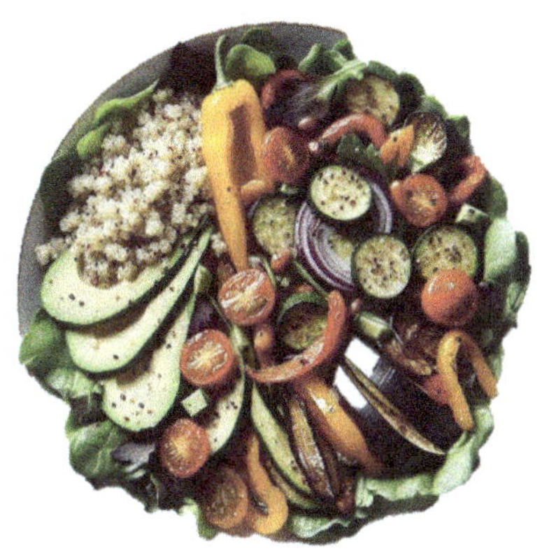

Quinoa Salad with Roasted Vegetables:

Ingredients:

- o 1 cup quinoa, rinsed, and cooked
- o 2 cups water or vegetable broth
- o 2 cups mixed vegetables
- o 2 tablespoons olive oil
- o Salt and pepper to taste
- o 1/4 cup chopped fresh herbs
- o Juice of 1 lemon

Instructions:

- ✓ Preheat the oven to 400°F (200°C).
- ✓ In an average-sized saucepan, bring water or vegetable broth to a boil. Add quinoa, reduce heat to low, cover, and simmer for 15-20 minutes until quinoa is cooked and liquid is absorbed. Remove from heat and let cool.
- ✓ Meanwhile, toss mixed vegetables (bell peppers, zucchini, and cherry tomatoes) with olive oil, salt, and pepper on a baking sheet.
- ✓ Roast in the preheated oven for 20-25 minutes, until vegetables are tender and slightly caramelized.
- ✓ In a large bowl, combine cooked quinoa, roasted vegetables, chopped fresh herbs (parsley or cilantro), and lemon juice. Toss to combine.
- ✓ Serve it warm or at room temperature.

Grilled Eggplant with Balsamic Glaze:

Ingredients:

- o 1 large eggplant, sliced into rounds
- o 2 tablespoons olive oil
- o Salt and pepper to taste
- o Balsamic glaze for drizzling

Instructions:

- ✓ Over medium-high heat, preheat the grill or the grill pan.
- ✓ Coat the eggplant slices with olive oil and season with salt and pepper.
- ✓ Grill eggplant slices for 4-5 minutes on each side, until tender and grill marks appear.
- ✓ Remove from the grill and arrange on a serving platter.
- ✓ Drizzle with balsamic glaze before serving.

Greek Yogurt Veggie Dip:

Ingredients:

- o 1 cup Greek yogurt
- o 1/4 cup finely chopped cucumber
- o 1/4 cup finely chopped red bell pepper
- o 1 tablespoon chopped fresh dill
- o 1 tablespoon lemon juice
- o 1 clove garlic, minced
- o Salt and pepper to taste

Instructions:

- ✓ In a bowl, combine Greek yogurt, chopped cucumber, chopped red bell pepper, chopped

fresh dill, lemon juice, minced garlic, salt, and pepper.
- ✓ Mix well until combined.
- ✓ Serve chilled with fresh vegetable sticks for dipping.

Roasted Garlic and Herb Chickpeas:

Ingredients:

- o 2 cups cooked chickpeas
- o 2 tablespoons olive oil
- o 2 cloves garlic, minced
- o 1 teaspoon dried thyme
- o 1 teaspoon dried rosemary
- o Salt and pepper to taste

Instructions:

- ✓ Preheat the oven to 200°C (400°F) and line a baking sheet with parchment paper.
- ✓ In a bowl, toss the cooked chickpeas with olive oil, minced garlic, dried thyme, dried rosemary, salt, and pepper until evenly coated.
- ✓ Gently spread the chickpeas in a single layer on the prepared baking sheet.

✓ Roast for 25–30 minutes, shaking the pan halfway through, until the chickpeas are crispy.
✓ Take it out of the oven and allow it to cool slightly before serving.

Cucumber Sushi Rolls:

Ingredients:

- 2 large cucumbers
- 1 cup cooked quinoa
- 1/2 avocado, sliced
- 1/2 red bell pepper, thinly sliced
- 1/4 cup shredded carrots
- 1/4 cup sliced cucumber
- 2 tablespoons rice vinegar
- 1 tablespoon honey or maple syrup
- Soy sauce for dipping

Instructions:

✓ Using a vegetable peeler, peel the cucumbers lengthwise into thin strips.
✓ Lay out cucumber strips on a flat surface.
✓ Spread cooked quinoa evenly over each cucumber strip, leaving a small border at the edges.

- ✓ Place avocado slices, red bell pepper slices, shredded carrots, and sliced cucumber on top of the quinoa.
- ✓ Roll up the cucumber strips tightly, securing with toothpicks if needed.
- ✓ In a small bowl, whisk together rice vinegar and honey or maple syrup.
- ✓ Drizzle the sushi rolls with the rice vinegar mixture.
- ✓ Serve with soy sauce for dipping.

Roasted Radishes:

Ingredients:

- o 1 bunch radishes, trimmed and halved
- o 1 tablespoon olive oil
- o Salt and pepper to taste

Instructions:

- ✓ Preheat the oven to 400°F (200°C).
- ✓ In a bowl, toss the radish halves with olive oil, salt, and pepper until evenly coated.
- ✓ Spread the radishes on a baking sheet lined with parchment paper.
- ✓ Roast for an average of 15–20 minutes, or until tender and slightly caramelized.
- ✓ Serve it hot as a delicious and nutritious snack or side dish.

Avocado and Tomato Salsa:

Ingredients:

- o 2 ripe avocados, diced
- o 1 cup cherry tomatoes, quartered
- o 1/4 cup red onion, finely chopped
- o 1 jalapeño, seeded and finely chopped
- o Juice of 1 lime
- o 2 tablespoons chopped fresh cilantro
- o Salt and pepper to taste

Instructions:

- ✓ In a bowl, combine diced avocados, quartered cherry tomatoes, finely chopped red onion, chopped jalapeño, lime juice, and chopped cilantro.
- ✓ Season with salt and pepper, to taste.
- ✓ Toss all the ingredients evenly until well combined.
- ✓ Serve immediately with whole grain tortilla chips or as a topping for grilled chicken or fish.

Roasted Beet and Walnut Salad:

Ingredients:

- o 3 medium beets, peeled and diced

- o 1 tablespoon olive oil
- o Salt and pepper to taste
- o 1/4 cup walnuts, chopped
- o 2 cups mixed salad greens
- o 2 tablespoons balsamic vinegar

Instructions:

- ✓ Preheat the oven to 400°F (200°C).
- ✓ In a bowl, toss the diced beets with olive oil, salt, and pepper until evenly coated.
- ✓ Carefully spread the beets on a baking sheet lined with parchment paper.
- ✓ Roast for an average of 25–30 minutes, or until tender and caramelized.
- ✓ In a dry skillet, toast the chopped walnuts over medium heat for 3–4 minutes, or until lightly golden and fragrant.
- ✓ In a large bowl, combine the roasted beets, toasted walnuts, and mixed salad greens.
- ✓ Drizzle with balsamic vinegar and toss gently to combine.
- ✓ Serve immediately as a flavorful and nutritious side salad.

Tuna and Cucumber Bites:

Ingredients:

- o 1 cucumber, sliced into rounds
- o 1 can (5 ounces) tuna, drained
- o 2 tablespoons Greek yogurt
- o 1 tablespoon lemon juice
- o 1 tablespoon chopped fresh dill
- o Salt and pepper to taste

Instructions:

- ✓ In a bowl, combine drained tuna, Greek yogurt, lemon juice, chopped fresh dill, salt, and pepper.
- ✓ Mix until all the ingredients are evenly incorporated or combined.
- ✓ Place cucumber rounds on a serving platter.
- ✓ Gently top each cucumber round with a spoonful of the tuna mixture.
- ✓ Serve immediately as a refreshing and protein-packed snack.

Cilantro Lime Coleslaw:

Ingredients:

- o 4 cups shredded cabbage (green or purple)
- o 1/4 cup chopped fresh cilantro
- o 2 tablespoons olive oil

- o   Juice of 2 limes
- o   1 tablespoon honey or maple syrup
- o   Salt and pepper to taste

Instructions:

- ✓ In a large bowl, combine shredded cabbage and chopped cilantro.
- ✓ In a small bowl, whisk together olive oil, lime juice, honey or maple syrup, salt, and pepper to make the dressing.
- ✓ Carefully pour the dressing over the cabbage mixture and toss until well-coated.
- ✓ Let the coleslaw sit for at least 10 minutes to allow the flavors to meld.
- ✓ Serve chilled as a refreshing and tangy side dish.

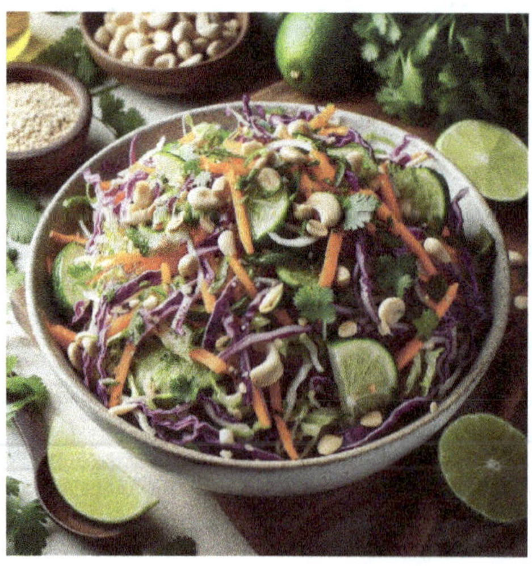

CHAPTER 9

Green Detox Smoothies

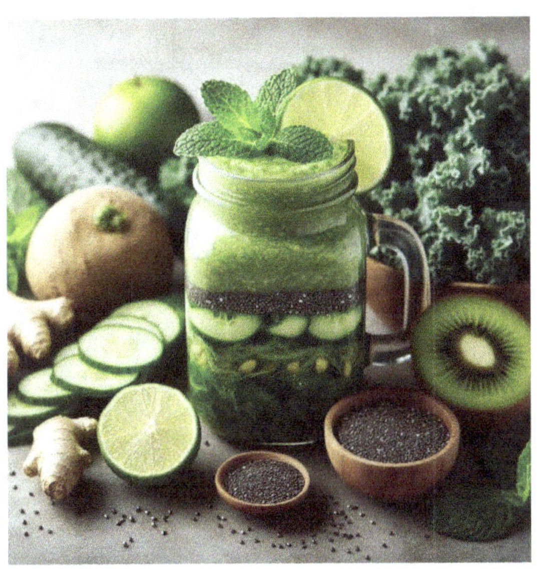

Spinach and Pineapple Detox Smoothie:

Ingredients:

- o 2 cups fresh spinach, washed
- o 1 cup chopped pineapple
- o 1/2 cucumber, peeled and chopped
- o 1 tablespoon fresh ginger, grated
- o 1 tablespoon lemon juice
- o 1 cup coconut water

Instructions:

- ✓ Place spinach, pineapple, cucumber, ginger, lemon juice, and coconut water in a blender.
- ✓ Blend until smooth and creamy.
- ✓ Pour into glasses and serve immediately.

Kale and Kiwi Detox Smoothie:

Ingredients:

- o 1 cup chopped kale leaves
- o 2 kiwis, peeled and chopped
- o 1/2 cup cucumber, chopped
- o 1/2 green apple, chopped
- o 1 tablespoon chia seeds
- o 1 cup coconut water

Instructions:

- ✓ Combine kale, kiwi, cucumber, apple, chia seeds, and coconut water in a blender.
- ✓ Blend until smooth and creamy.
- ✓ Pour into glasses and enjoy!

Green Detox Smoothie with Celery and Pear:

Ingredients:

- 2 cups spinach
- 2 stalks celery, chopped
- 1 pear, cored and chopped
- 1/2 cucumber, chopped
- 1 tablespoon fresh parsley
- 1 tablespoon lemon juice
- 1 cup almond milk (unsweetened)

Instructions:

- Add spinach, celery, pear, cucumber, parsley, lemon juice, and almond milk to a blender.
- Blend until smooth and creamy.
- Pour into glasses and serve immediately.

Avocado and Spinach Detox Smoothie:

Ingredients:

- 1 ripe avocado
- 2 cups fresh spinach
- 1/2 cup chopped cucumber
- 1/2 cup chopped pineapple
- 1 tablespoon fresh mint leaves
- 1 tablespoon lime juice

o   1 cup coconut water

Instructions:

- ✓ Combine avocado, spinach, cucumber, pineapple, mint leaves, lime juice, and coconut water in a blender.
- ✓ Blend until smooth and creamy.
- ✓ Pour into glasses and enjoy!

Green Detox Smoothie with Cucumber and Mint:

Ingredients:

o   1 cup chopped cucumber
o   1 cup spinach
o   1/2 cup chopped pineapple
o   1/2 green apple, chopped
o   1 tablespoon fresh mint leaves
o   1 tablespoon lime juice
o   1 cup coconut water

Instructions:

- ✓ Place cucumber, spinach, pineapple, apple, mint leaves, lime juice, and coconut water in a blender.
- ✓ Blend until smooth and creamy.
- ✓ Pour into glasses and serve immediately.

Kale and Banana Detox Smoothie:

Ingredients:

- o 2 cups chopped kale leaves
- o 1 banana
- o 1/2 cup chopped cucumber
- o 1 tablespoon fresh ginger, grated
- o 1 tablespoon chia seeds
- o 1 cup almond milk (unsweetened)

Instructions:

- ✓ Add kale, banana, cucumber, ginger, chia seeds, and almond milk to a blender.
- ✓ Blend until smooth and creamy.
- ✓ Pour into glasses and enjoy!

Green Detox Smoothie with Spinach and Mango:

Ingredients:

- o 2 cups fresh spinach
- o 1 cup chopped mango
- o 1/2 cup chopped cucumber
- o 1 tablespoon fresh ginger, grated
- o 1 tablespoon lemon juice
- o 1 cup coconut water

Instructions:

- ✓ Combine spinach, mango, cucumber, ginger, lemon juice, and coconut water in a blender.
- ✓ Blend until smooth and creamy.
- ✓ Pour into glasses and enjoy!

Green Goddess Detox Smoothie:

Ingredients:

- o 1 cup kale
- o 1/2 cup cucumber, chopped
- o 1/2 avocado
- o 1/2 cup pineapple chunks
- o 1 tablespoon fresh mint leaves

- o   1 tablespoon lime juice
- o   1 cup coconut water or water

Instructions:

- ✓ Wash the kale and cucumber thoroughly.
- ✓ Pit and scoop out the avocado.
- ✓ Chop the cucumber into smaller pieces after peeling.
- ✓ In a blender, combine all the ingredients.
- ✓ Blend until smooth.
- ✓ Pour into glasses and serve immediately.

Green Detox Smoothie with Spinach and Orange:

Ingredients:

- o   2 cups fresh spinach
- o   1 orange, peeled and chopped
- o   1/2 cup chopped cucumber
- o   1/2 green apple, chopped
- o   1 tablespoon fresh mint leaves
- o   1 tablespoon lemon juice
- o   1 cup coconut water

Instructions:

- ✓ Add spinach, orange, cucumber, apple, mint leaves, lemon juice, and coconut water to a blender.
- ✓ Blend until smooth and creamy.
- ✓ Pour into glasses and enjoy!

Green Detox Hydration Smoothie:

Ingredients:

- o 2 cups spinach
- o 1 cucumber, chopped
- o 1/2 cup celery, chopped
- o 1/2 cup green grapes
- o 1 tablespoon parsley leaves
- o 1 tablespoon lemon juice
- o 1 cup coconut water or water

Instructions:

- ✓ Wash the spinach, cucumber, celery, and grapes thoroughly.
- ✓ Chop the cucumber and celery into smaller pieces.
- ✓ In a blender, combine all the ingredients.
- ✓ Blend until smooth.
- ✓ Pour into glasses and serve immediately.

Detoxifying Green Veggie Smoothie:

Ingredients:

- o 1 cup broccoli florets
- o 1/2 cup celery, chopped
- o 1/2 cup cucumber, chopped
- o 1/2 cup green apple, chopped
- o 1 tablespoon fresh parsley leaves
- o 1 tablespoon lemon juice
- o 1 cup coconut water or water

Instructions:

- ✓ Wash the broccoli, celery, cucumber, and apple thoroughly.
- ✓ Chop the celery, cucumber, and apple into smaller pieces.
- ✓ In a blender, combine all the ingredients.
- ✓ Blend until smooth.
- ✓ Pour into glasses and serve immediately.

CONCLUSION

Endomorph Diet for Beginners serves as a guiding light for those embarking on a journey towards better health and wellness. Throughout this book, we've explored the intricacies of the endomorph body type and provided valuable insights into crafting a sustainable and effective dietary approach tailored specifically to its needs. From understanding the fundamentals of nutrition to practical meal planning, from incorporating delicious recipes to embracing lifestyle changes, this book equips you with the knowledge and tools necessary to thrive on your endomorph journey.

As you close these pages, remember that transformation is not just about shedding pounds alone but also about nourishing your body, mind, and spirit. Embrace the power within you to make informed choices, prioritize self-care, and cultivate a positive relationship with food and fitness. Let this book be your companion, guiding you towards a path of empowerment, vitality, and lasting transformation.

——John Milton Doe

30 DAYS MEAL PLAN

Day 1:

- ➢ **Breakfast:** Omelet with spinach and cheese
- ➢ **Lunch:** Grilled Chicken Salad
- ➢ **Dinner:** Baked Lemon Herb Chicken
- ➢ **Dessert:** Baked Apples with Cinnamon
- ➢ **Snack/Side Dish:** Quinoa Salad with Roasted Vegetables

Day 2:

- ➢ **Breakfast:** Greek yogurt with berries & nuts
- ➢ **Lunch:** Black Bean Stuffed Bell Peppers with Quinoa
- ➢ **Dinner:** Garlic Shrimp Pasta
- ➢ **Dessert:** Banana Oatmeal Cookies
- ➢ **Snack/Side Dish:** Grilled Eggplant with Balsamic Glaze

Day 3:

- ➢ **Breakfast:** Quinoa porridge
- ➢ **Lunch:** Salmon and Asparagus Foil Packets
- ➢ **Dinner:** Vegetable and Chickpea Curry
- ➢ **Dessert:** Dark Chocolate Avocado Mousse
- ➢ **Snack/Side Dish:** Greek Yogurt Veggie Dip

Day 4:

- ➢ **Breakfast:** Avocado toast with eggs and bacon
- ➢ **Lunch:** Turkey and Avocado Wrap
- ➢ **Dinner:** Eggplant Parmesan
- ➢ **Dessert:** Coconut Mango Sorbet
- ➢ **Snack/Side Dish:** Roasted Garlic and Herb Chickpeas

Day 5:

- ➢ **Breakfast:** Smoothie bowl with granola and fruits
- ➢ **Lunch:** Lentil and Vegetable Soup
- ➢ **Dinner:** Turkey Meatballs with Zucchini Noodles
- ➢ **Dessert:** Almond Flour Banana Bread
- ➢ **Snack/Side Dish:** Cucumber Sushi Rolls

Day 6:

- ➢ **Breakfast:** Chia pudding with coconut and pineapple
- ➢ **Lunch:** Veggie and Hummus Sandwich
- ➢ **Dinner:** Baked Teriyaki Chicken
- ➢ **Dessert:** Baked Pears with Cinnamon and Walnuts
- ➢ **Snack/Side Dish**: Avocado and Tomato Salsa

Day 7:

- ➢ **Breakfast:** Egg muffins with ham and cheese
- ➢ **Lunch:** Chicken and Vegetable Stir-Fry
- ➢ **Dinner:** Moroccan Chickpea Tagine
- ➢ **Dessert:** Raspberry Chia Jam
- ➢ **Snack/Side Dish:** Roasted Beet and Walnut Salad

Day 8:

- ➢ **Breakfast:** Salmon and cream cheese bagel
- ➢ **Lunch:** Shrimp and Avocado Salad
- ➢ **Dinner:** Thai Peanut Chicken Lettuce Wraps
- ➢ **Dessert:** Cinnamon Baked Pear Chips
- ➢ Snack/Side Dish: Tuna and Cucumber Bites

Day 9:

- ➢ **Breakfast:** Almond butter and banana waffles
- ➢ **Lunch:** Veggie and Quinoa Stuffed Sweet Potatoes
- ➢ **Dinner:** Salmon and Asparagus Foil Packs
- ➢ **Dessert:** Lemon Poppy Seed Muffins
- ➢ **Snack/Side** Dish: Cilantro Lime Coleslaw

Day 10:

- ➢ **Breakfast:** Omelet with spinach and cheese
- ➢ **Lunch:** Grilled Chicken Salad
- ➢ **Dinner:** Baked Lemon Herb Chicken
- ➢ **Dessert:** Baked Apples with Cinnamon
- ➢ **Snack/Side Dish:** Quinoa Salad with Roasted Vegetables

Day 11:

- ➢ **Breakfast:** Greek yogurt with berries and nuts
- ➢ **Lunch:** Black Bean Stuffed Bell Peppers with Quinoa
- ➢ **Dinner:** Garlic Shrimp Pasta
- ➢ **Dessert:** Banana Oatmeal Cookies
- ➢ **Snack/Side Dish:** Grilled Eggplant with Balsamic Glaze

Day 12:

- ➢ **Breakfast:** Quinoa porridge
- ➢ **Lunch:** Salmon and Asparagus Foil Packets
- ➢ **Dinner:** Vegetable and Chickpea Curry
- ➢ **Dessert:** Dark Chocolate Avocado Mousse
- ➢ **Snack/Side Dish:** Greek Yogurt Veggie Dip

Day 13:

- **Breakfast:** Avocado toast with eggs and bacon
- **Lunch:** Turkey and Avocado Wrap
- **Dinner:** Eggplant Parmesan
- **Dessert:** Coconut Mango Sorbet
- **Snack/Side Dish:** Roasted Garlic and Herb Chickpeas

Day 14:

- **Breakfast:** Smoothie bowl with granola and fruits
- **Lunch:** Lentil and Vegetable Soup
- **Dinner:** Turkey Meatballs with Zucchini Noodles
- **Dessert:** Almond Flour Banana Bread
- **Snack/Side Dish:** Cucumber Sushi Rolls

Day 15:

- **Breakfast:** Cottage cheese pancakes
- **Lunch:** Tuna Salad Lettuce Wraps
- **Dinner:** Stuffed Portobello Mushrooms
- **Dessert:** Protein-Packed Chocolate Peanut Butter Balls
- **Snack/Side Dish:** Roasted Radishes

> - **Breakfast:** Chia pudding with coconut and pineapple
> - **Lunch:** Veggie and Hummus Sandwich
> - **Dinner:** Baked Teriyaki Chicken
> - **Dessert:** Baked Pears with Cinnamon and Walnuts
> - **Snack/Side Dish:** Avocado and Tomato Salsa

Day 17:

> - **Breakfast:** Egg muffins with ham and cheese
> - **Lunch:** Chicken and Vegetable Stir-Fry
> - **Dinner:** Moroccan Chickpea Tagine
> - **Dessert:** Raspberry Chia Jam
> - **Snack/Side Dish:** Roasted Beet and Walnut Salad

Day 18:

> - **Breakfast:** Salmon and cream cheese bagel
> - **Lunch:** Shrimp and Avocado Salad
> - **Dinner:** Thai Peanut Chicken Lettuce Wraps
> - **Dessert:** Cinnamon Baked Pear Chips
> - **Snack/Side Dish:** Tuna and Cucumber Bites

Day 19:

- ➤ **Breakfast:** Almond butter and banana waffles
- ➤ **Lunch:** Veggie and Quinoa Stuffed Sweet Potatoes
- ➤ **Dinner:** Salmon and Asparagus Foil Packs
- ➤ **Dessert:** Lemon Poppy Seed Muffins
- ➤ **Snack/Side Dish:** Cilantro Lime Coleslaw

Day 20:

- ➤ **Breakfast:** Omelet with spinach and cheese
- ➤ **Lunch:** Grilled Chicken Salad
- ➤ **Dinner:** Baked Lemon Herb Chicken
- ➤ **Dessert:** Baked Apples with Cinnamon
- ➤ **Snack/Side Dish:** Quinoa Salad with Roasted Vegetables

Day 21:

- ➤ **Breakfast:** Greek yogurt with berries and nuts
- ➤ **Lunch:** Black Bean Stuffed Bell Peppers with Quinoa
- ➤ **Dinner:** Garlic Shrimp Pasta
- ➤ **Dessert:** Banana Oatmeal Cookies
- ➤ **Snack/Side Dish:** Grilled Eggplant with Balsamic Glaze

Day 22:

- ➤ **Breakfast:** Quinoa porridge
- ➤ **Lunch:** Salmon and Asparagus Foil Packets
- ➤ **Dinner:** Vegetable and Chickpea Curry
- ➤ **Dessert:** Dark Chocolate Avocado Mousse
- ➤ **Snack/Side Dish:** Greek Yogurt Veggie Dip

Day 23:

- ➤ **Breakfast:** Avocado toast with eggs and bacon
- ➤ **Lunch:** Turkey and Avocado Wrap
- ➤ **Dinner:** Eggplant Parmesan
- ➤ **Dessert:** Coconut Mango Sorbet
- ➤ **Snack/Side Dish:** Roasted Garlic and Herb Chickpeas

Day 24:

- ➤ **Breakfast:** Smoothie bowl with granola and fruits
- ➤ **Lunch:** Lentil and Vegetable Soup
- ➤ **Dinner:** Turkey Meatballs with Zucchini Noodles
- ➤ **Dessert:** Almond Flour Banana Bread
- ➤ **Snack/Side Dish:** Cucumber Sushi Rolls

Day 25:

- **Breakfast:** Cottage cheese pancakes
- **Lunch:** Tuna Salad Lettuce Wraps
- **Dinner:** Stuffed Portobello Mushrooms
- **Dessert:** Protein-Packed Chocolate Peanut Butter Balls
- **Snack/Side Dish:** Roasted Radishes

Day 26:

- **Breakfast:** Chia pudding with coconut and pineapple
- **Lunch:** Veggie and Hummus Sandwich
- **Dinner:** Baked Teriyaki Chicken
- **Dessert:** Baked Pears with Cinnamon and Walnuts
- **Snack/Side Dish:** Avocado and Tomato Salsa

Day 27:

- **Breakfast:** Egg muffins with ham and cheese
- **Lunch:** Chicken and Vegetable Stir-Fry
- **Dinner:** Moroccan Chickpea Tagine
- **Dessert:** Raspberry Chia Jam
- **Snack/Side Dish:** Roasted Beet and Walnut Salad

Day 28:

- ➢ Breakfast: Salmon and cream cheese bagel
- ➢ **Lunch:** Shrimp and Avocado Salad
- ➢ **Dinner:** Thai Peanut Chicken Lettuce Wraps
- ➢ **Dessert:** Cinnamon Baked Pear Chips
- ➢ **Snack/Side Dish:** Tuna and Cucumber Bites

Day 29:

- ➢ **Breakfast:** Almond butter and banana waffles
- ➢ **Lunch:** Veggie and Quinoa Stuffed Sweet Potatoes
- ➢ **Dinner:** Salmon and Asparagus Foil Packs
- ➢ **Dessert:** Lemon Poppy Seed Muffins
- ➢ **Snack/Side Dish:** Cilantro Lime Coleslaw

Day 30:

- ➢ **Breakfast:** Omelet with spinach and cheese
- ➢ **Lunch:** Grilled Chicken Salad
- ➢ **Dinner:** Baked Lemon Herb Chicken
- ➢ **Dessert:** Baked Apples with Cinnamon
- ➢ **Snack/Side Dish:** Quinoa Salad with Roasted Vegetables